Maya & Friends Visit the Acupuncturist

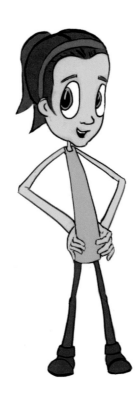

To learn more about Maya and her friends, and the world of acupuncture and Chinese medicine, visit:

acupuncturekidsbook.com

You can also get the eBook for your tablet or computer!

Thanks to Jason Robertson and Daniel Altschuler for their input, encouragement, and support in creating this book, and thank you to all of the instructors at SIOM for their dedication to teaching Chinese medicine.

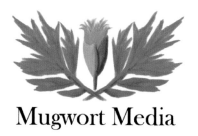

Mugwort Media

ISBN 978-0-9909184-2-4

Second Edition, December 2014

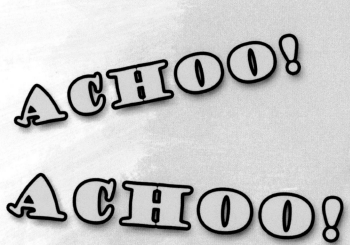

ACHOO!

ACHOO!

... went Maya's nose.

She felt a chill down to her toes.

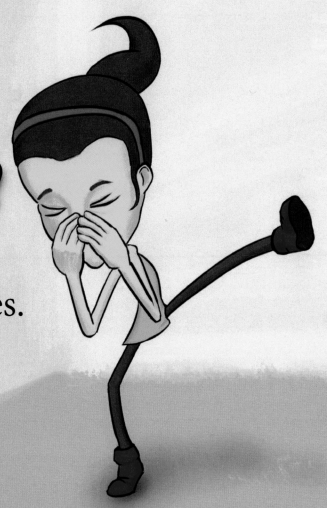

"Oh no!" said her friend Bobby Bear.
"Looks like you caught something in this cold air!"

She had chills, a fever, and her nose was runny.
Her throat was sore and her voice sounded funny.

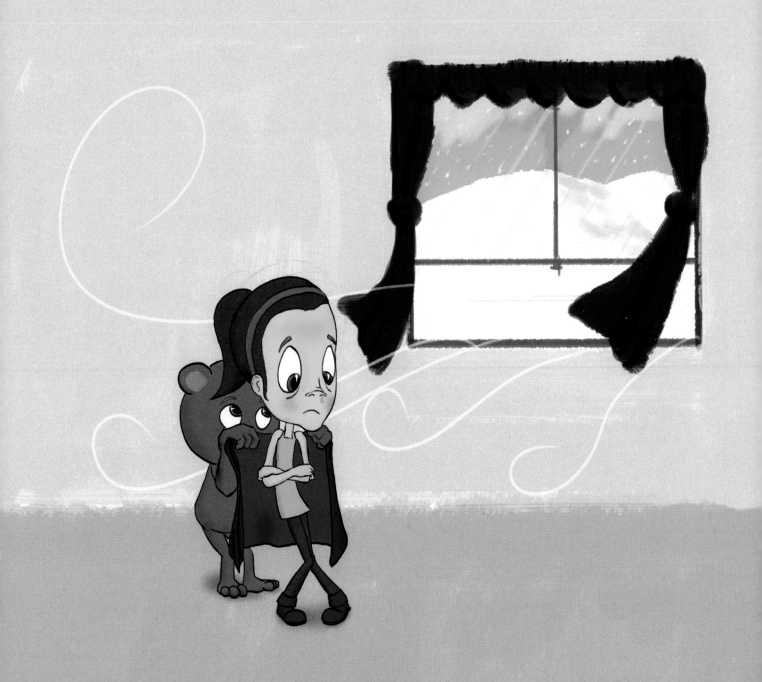

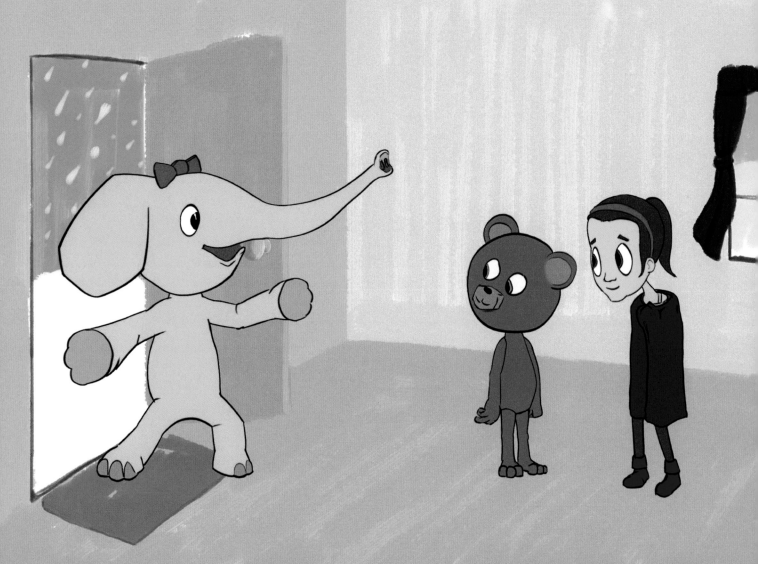

Ellie Elephant burst into the room,
"You're looking for help, I presume?"

"Why yes," said Maya, "Do you know who to call?"

"Dr. Meow—she's seen it all!"

"She uses acupuncture, herbs, and many techniques. She helped heal my trunk in just a few weeks."

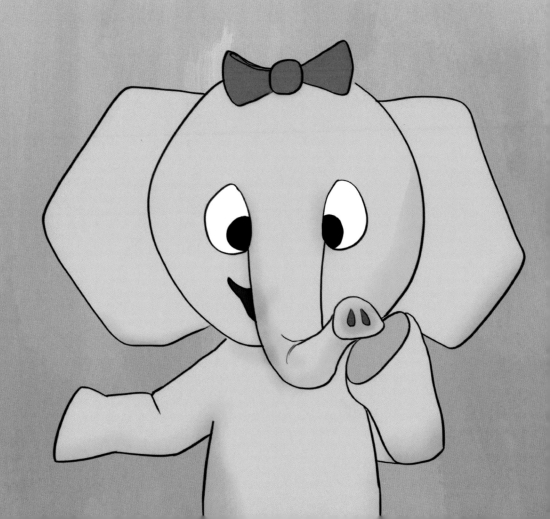

"That's it!" said Maya, "Let's pay her a visit!"
Bobby Bear exclaimed, "I wouldn't miss it!"

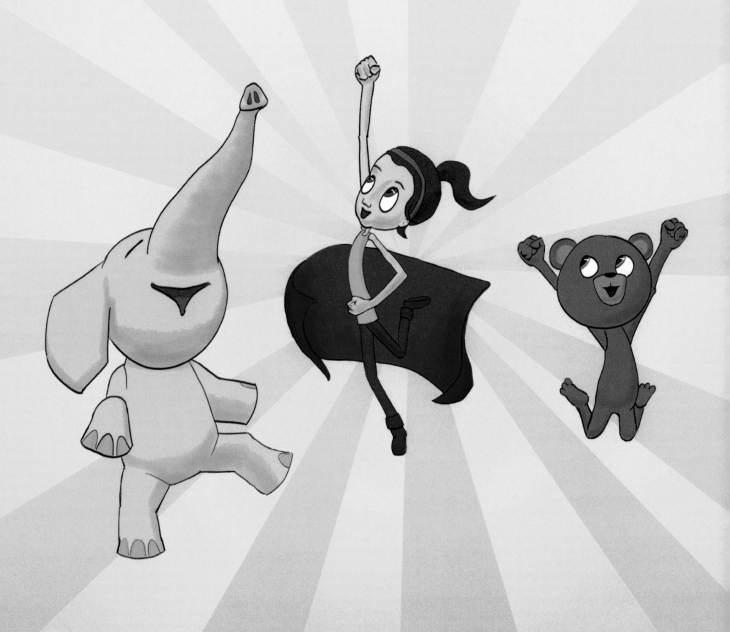

So they grabbed their **sled** and rode **away**,
To see the **acupuncturist** that very **day!**

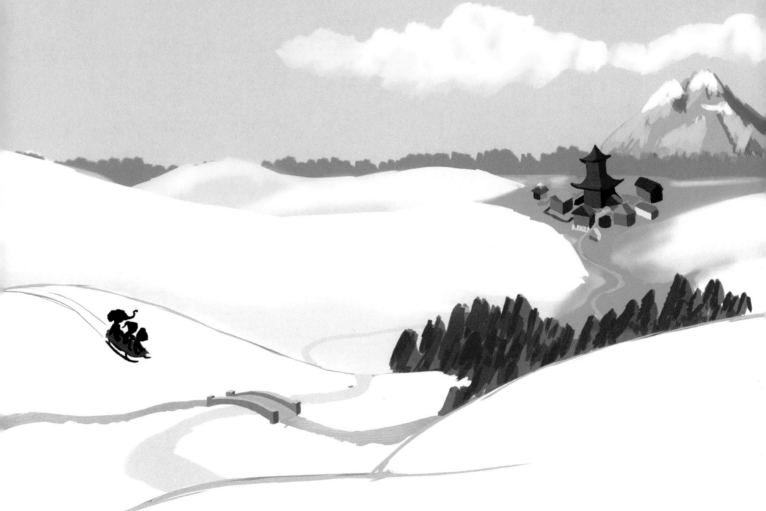

Over the **hills** and beyond the **stream**,
They traveled together as a **happy team.**

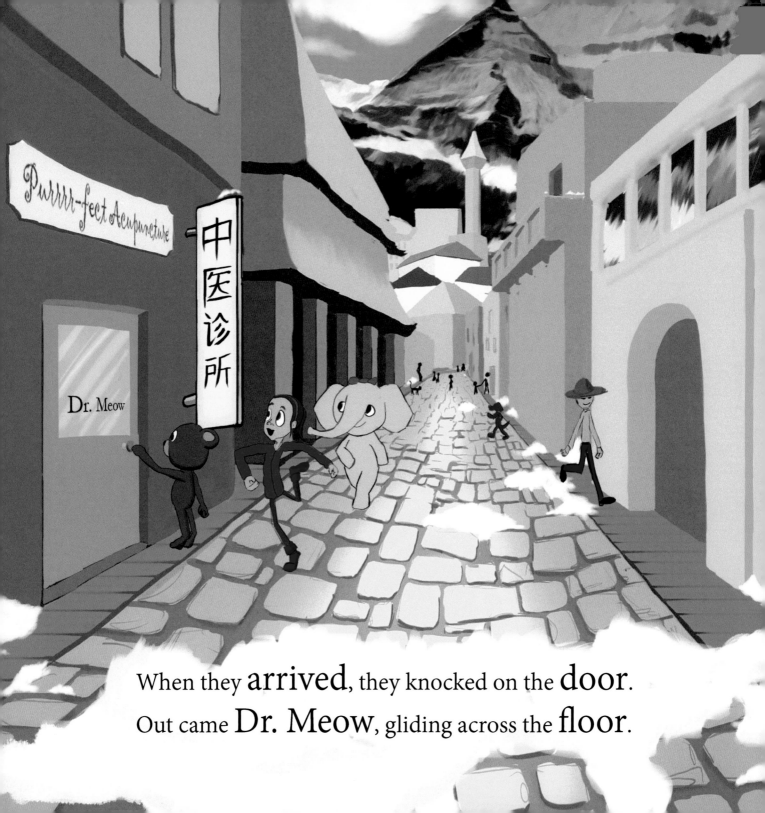

When they **arrived**, they knocked on the **door**.
Out came **Dr. Meow**, gliding across the **floor**.

"Welcome," she said. "What can I do for you?"

Maya pointed to her nose and out came an...

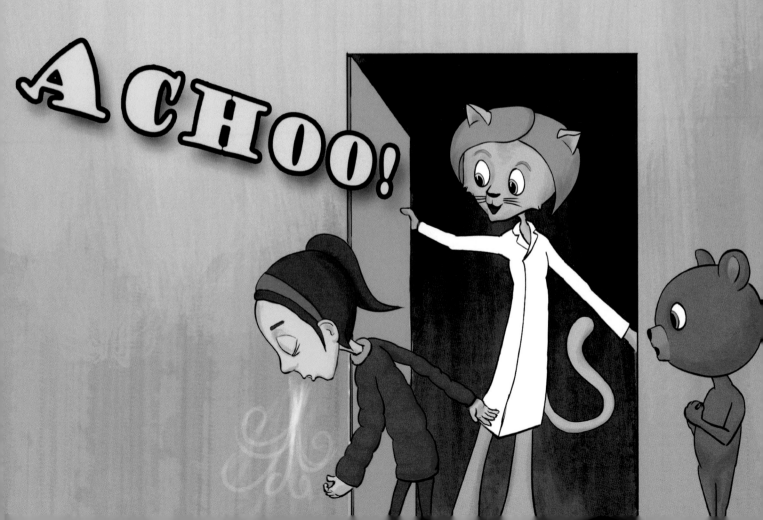

"Come right in, lie down, get nice and cozy.
Feel free to ask questions—that's not being nosy."

"Good," said Ellie. "I like to ask and explore.
My trunk always seems to want to know more!"

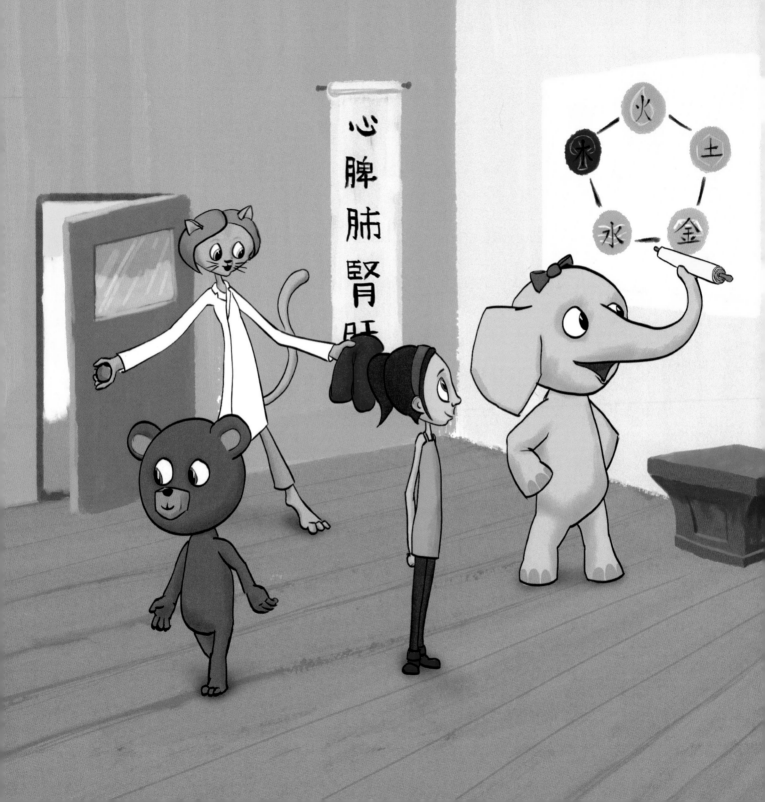

"First I will feel what your pulse has to say:
Does your body need rest, or does it want to play?"

"Then I will ask you to stick out your tongue,
As silly as that seems.
It gives me information on
Your body's patterns or themes..."

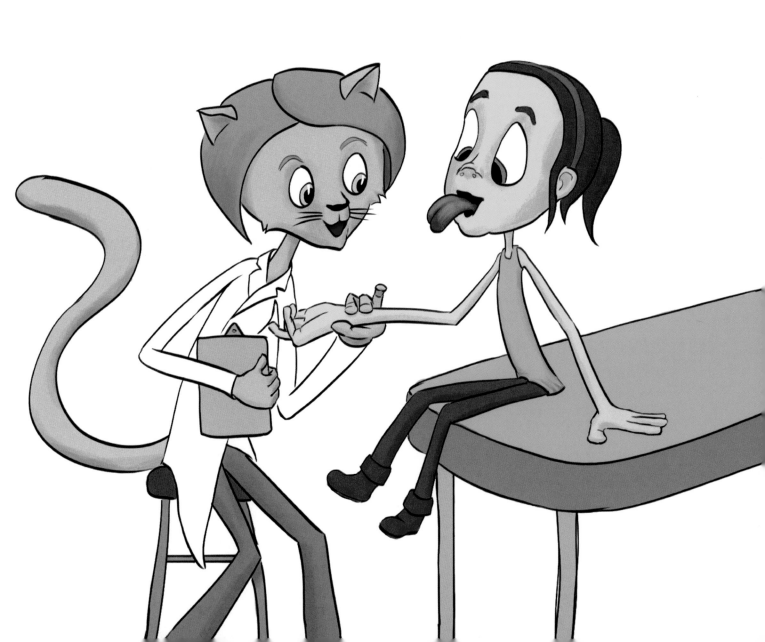

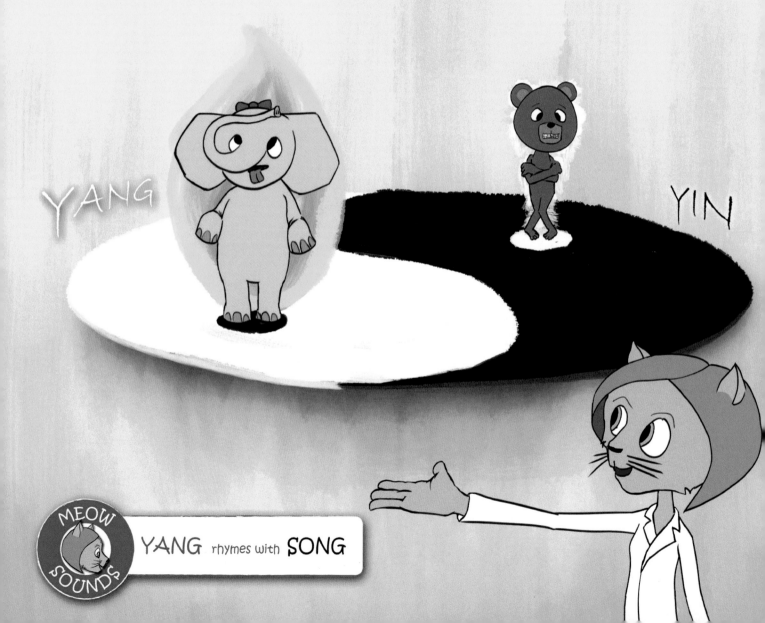

"Such as: Is there more **heat** or more **cold**, more **yang** or more **yin**? Is your body's **energy overflowing**, or is it running **thin**?"

YANG

YIN

MEOW SOUNDS

YANG rhymes with SONG

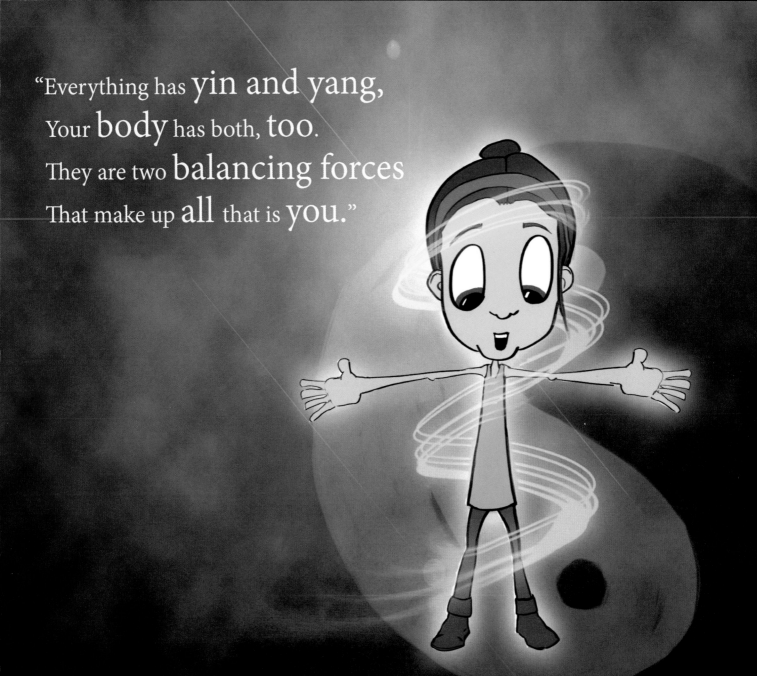

"Everything has yin and yang,
Your body has both, too.
They are two balancing forces
That make up all that is you."

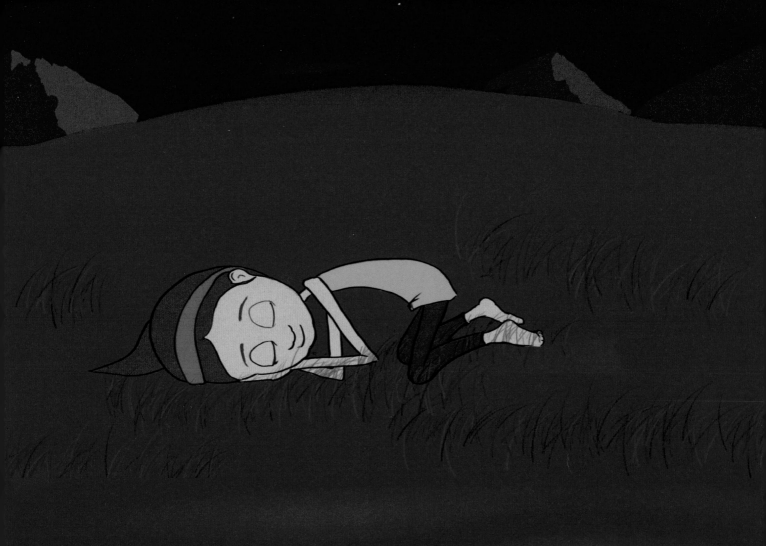

"When you go to sleep at night,
And the moon is shining bright,
The air feels cool as you sleep sound.
This is when yin is all around."

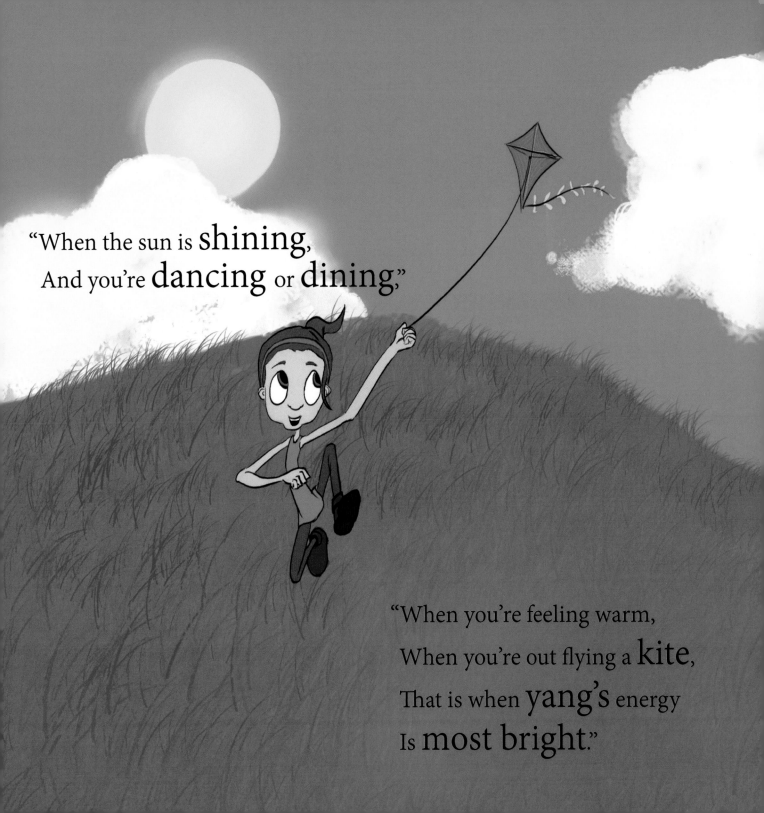

"When the sun is shining,
And you're dancing or dining,"

"When you're feeling warm,
When you're out flying a kite,
That is when yang's energy
Is most bright."

"It looks like you **caught** a **cold** in this chilly windy weather,

But not to worry—we can help get you **better.**"

"I have some **herbs** that you can **take** if you would like to try.

Of course I know that you may want to know **why.**"

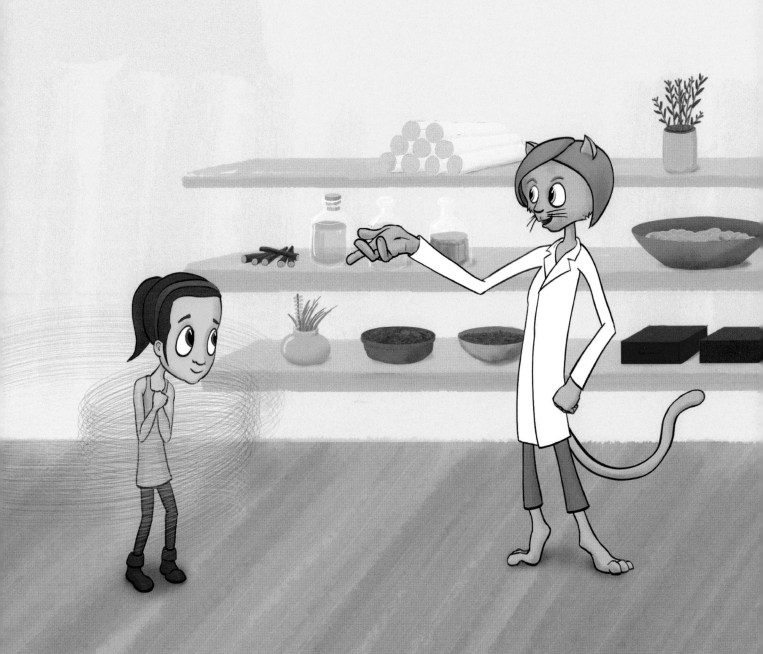

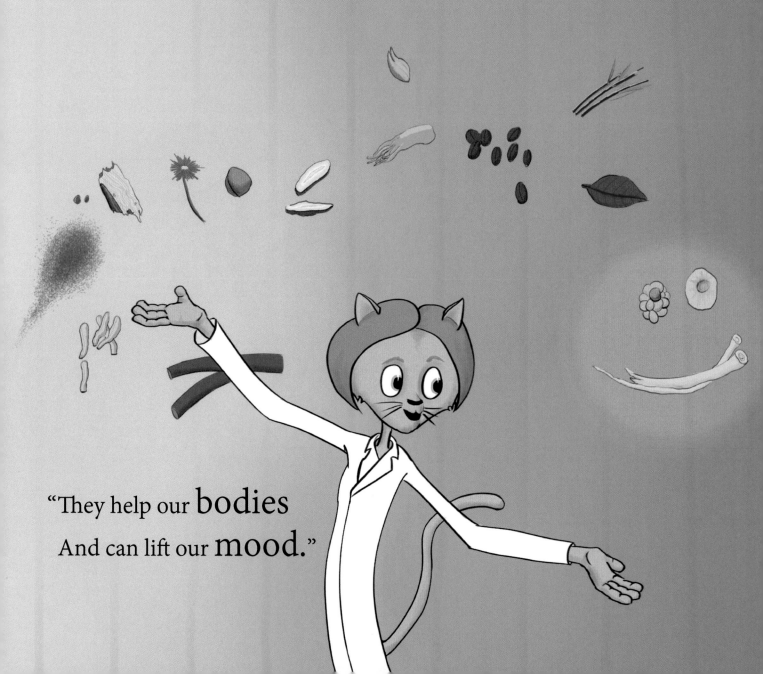

"Herbs are plants that are
Both medicine and food."

"They help our bodies
And can lift our mood."

"Here are some herbs for you to see.
Many are flowers, roots, berries, and leaves."

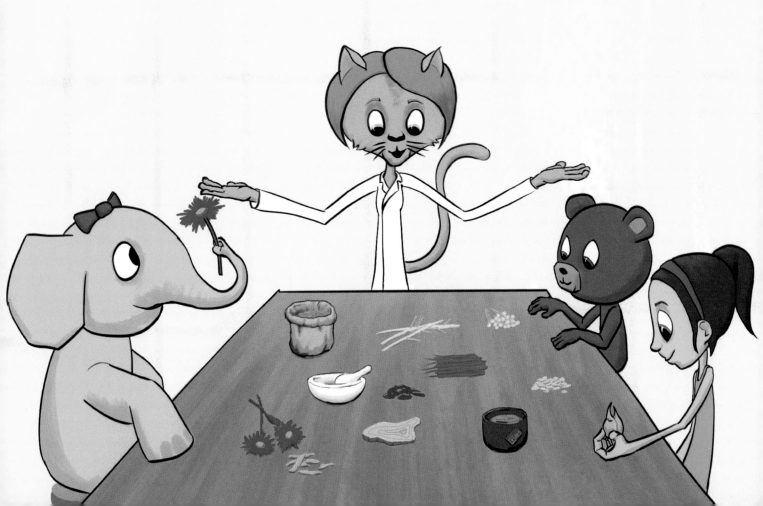

"Food can also be very important
For your body's qi.
Food is some of the best medicine
That there can be."

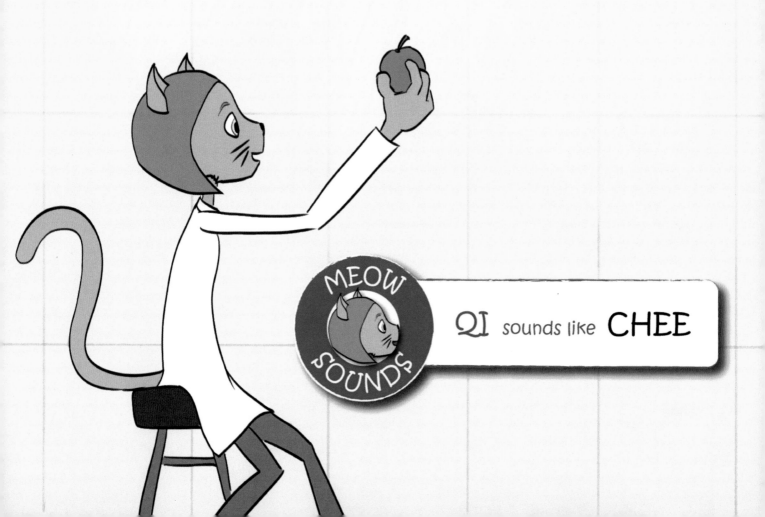

MEOW SOUNDS

QI sounds like CHEE

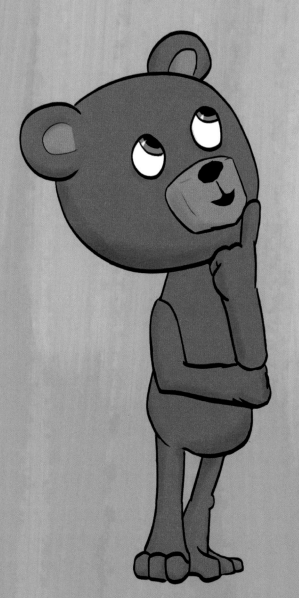

"What is qi?"
Asked Bobby Bear.
"Is it something in my body,
Or is it in the air?"

"Qi is energy. It is in your body and in the food you eat,
It is in your heart and it is in your feet."

"Qi flows through river-like channels bringing energy out and in.
You can imagine these channels when you look at your skin."

"Each channel is connected to an organ, such as your heart.
Many channels flow through each body part."

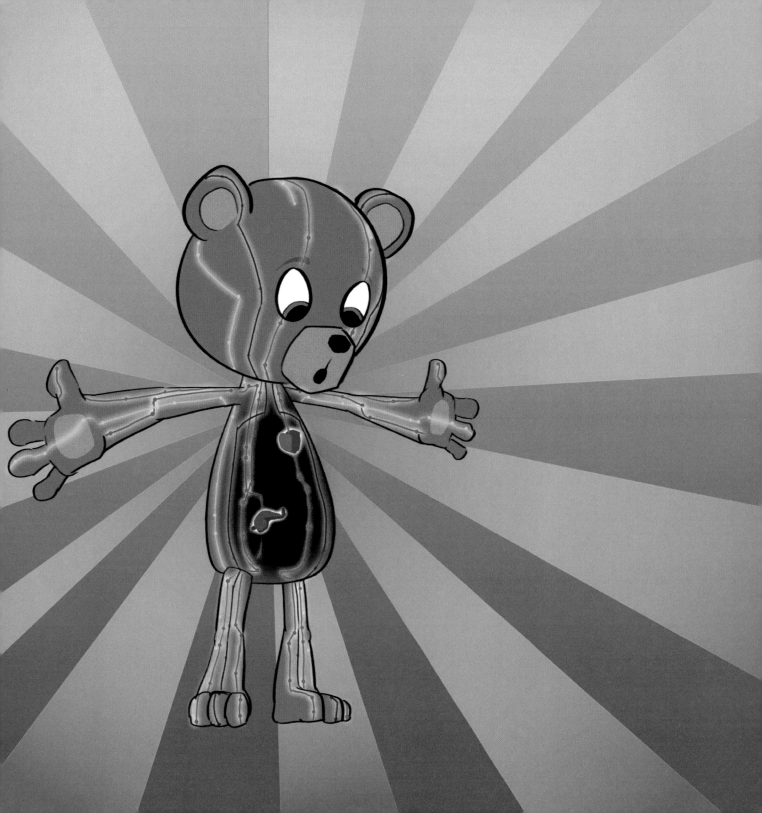

"I can gently press areas of your body
   Where these acupuncture channels flow.
   I can show you where they are
   So that you will know."

"This is called acupressure
   Because we press a certain point or line.
   It can make your tummy feel better
   Or your head or your spine."

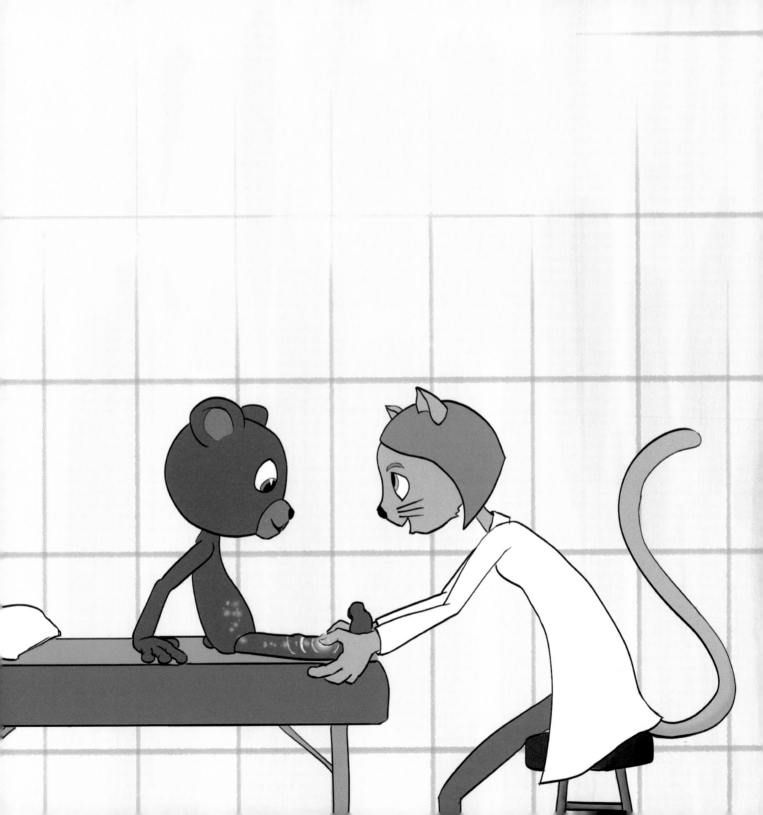

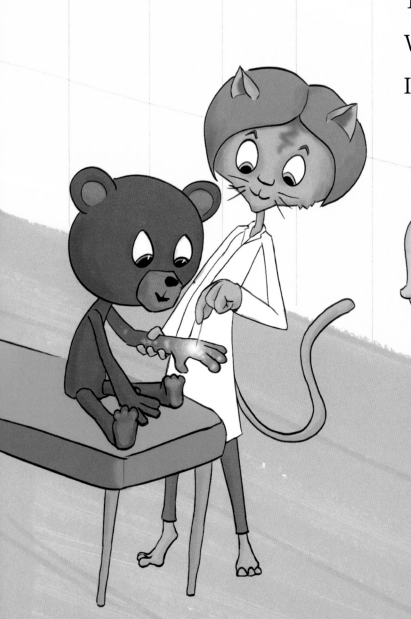

"I can also use a **special** needle
That is very **thin** and **light**.
When it touches your body
It makes everything **right**."

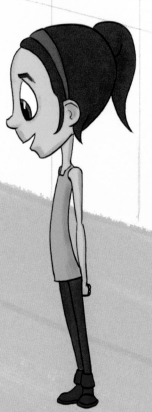

"We can place glass cups gently on your skin,
To help **soften** and **warm** any tension."

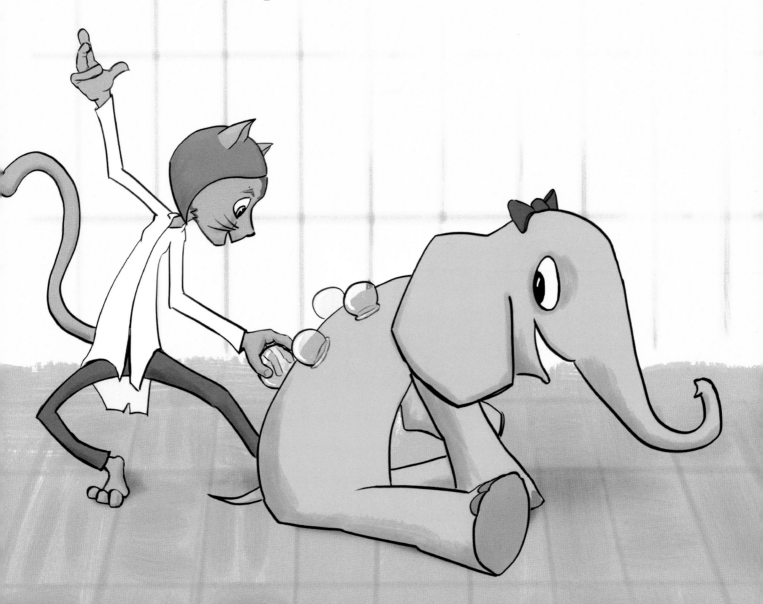

"Moxa is what we call a special warming technique. It works wonderfully if warmth is what you seek."

"It is made from the fuzz of the mugwort leaf. It feels very nice and can give great relief."

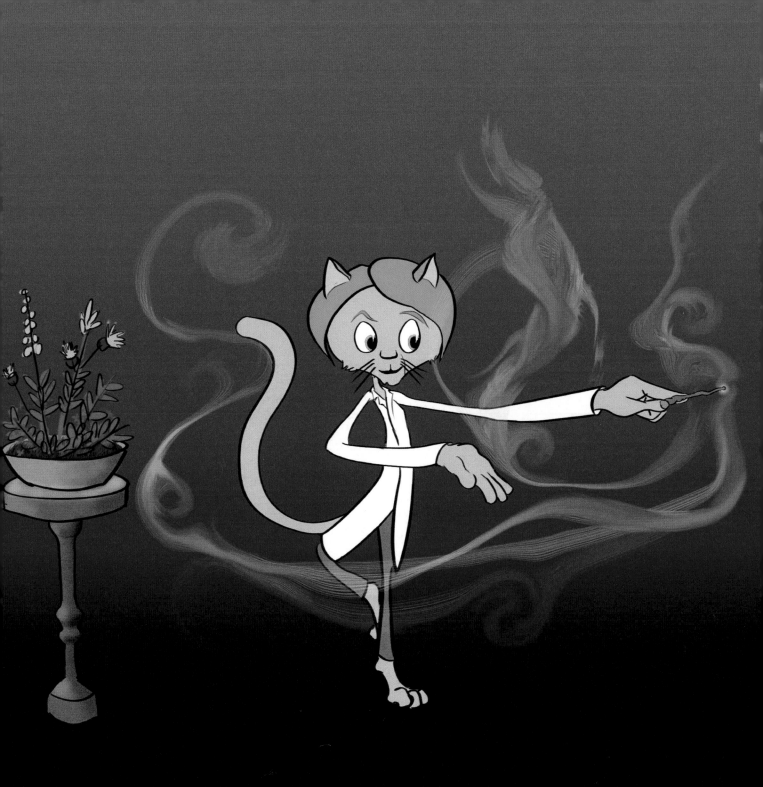

"As you can see, you have some choices of what we can do. Whatever happens to your body is up to you."

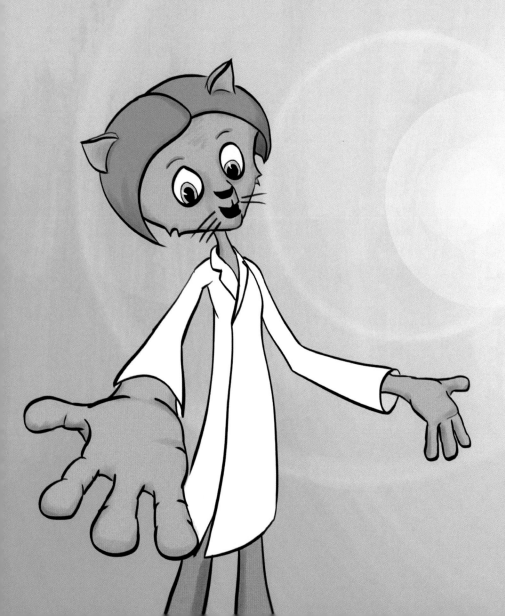

"Let's do **acupressure** on your lung channel,
Because your nose is stuffy."

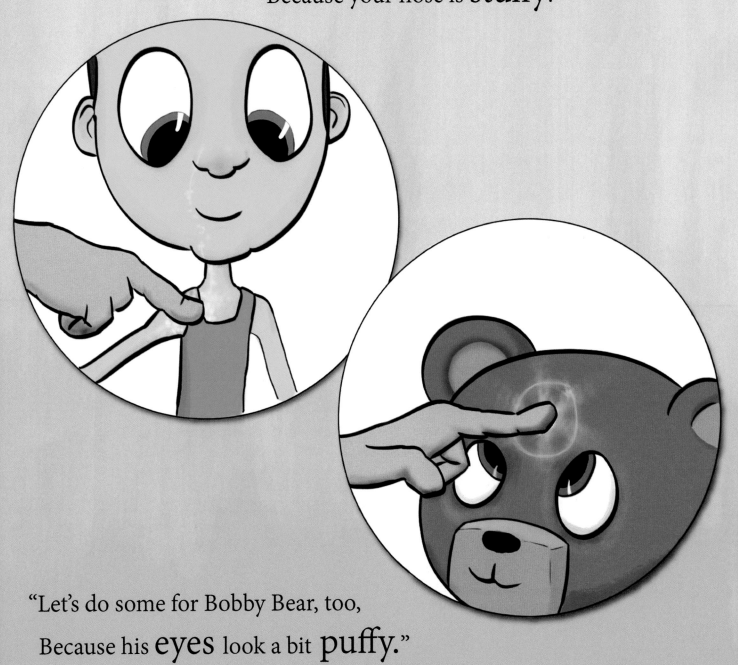

"Let's do some for Bobby Bear, too,
Because his **eyes** look a bit **puffy.**"

"Let's put some **herbs together**: Some flowers, twigs, and roots. You can drink it as a **flower tea** or mix it in with juice."

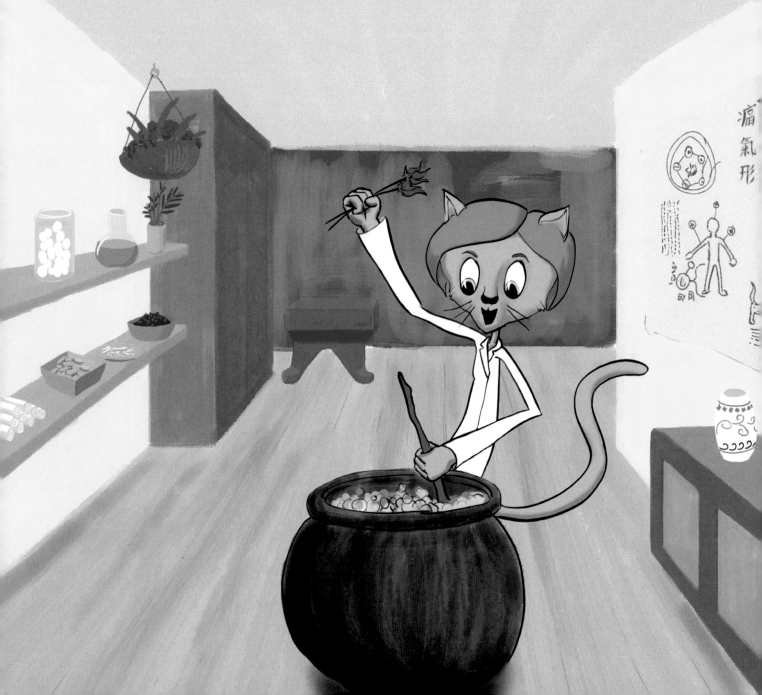

"Go home, **eat** some soup, and drink your **herbs** tonight.
Get a good night's **sleep** and tomorrow you should **feel all right**."

Maya put on her **jacket**
to keep cozy for the **ride**.

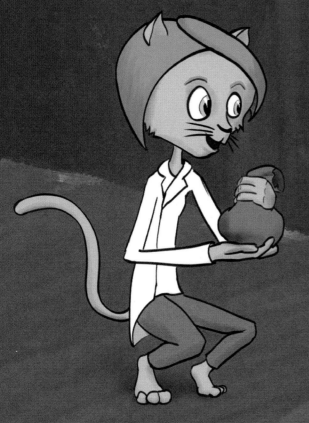
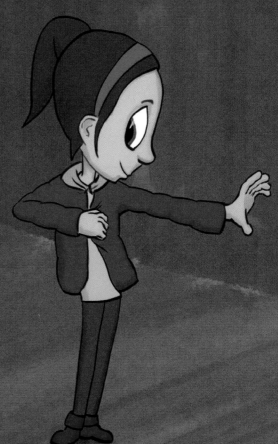

She wanted to **balance** yin and yang
and keep her **warmth inside**.

Dr. Meow waved goodbye
And the three set off on their way,
Thinking about the world around them
And all they learned today.

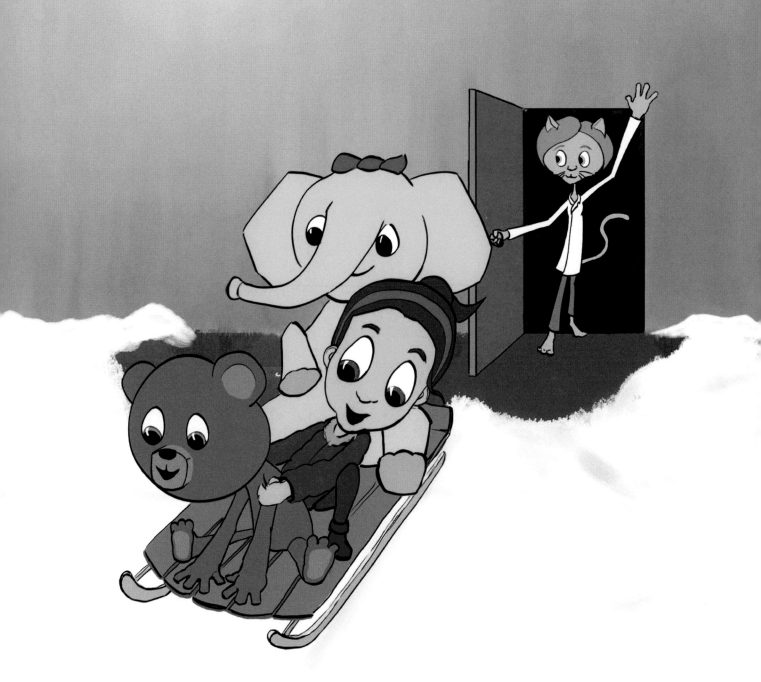

Ellie realized the fragrant scent of wood from the trees,
Smelled like the herbs in Dr. Meow's teas.

Bobby Bear noticed that lamp posts looked like needles in the street.
Their tops were glowing brightly like the moxa's warming heat.

Maya saw channels in the pathways that they sledded through.
She thought about the world around her that she is connected to.

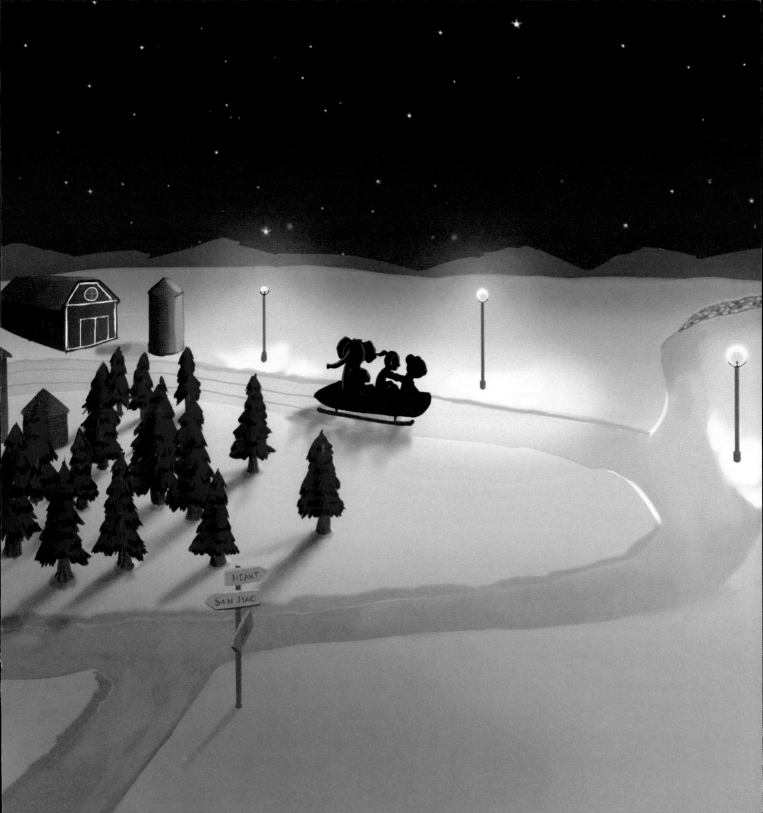

Across the stream and back over the hill,
Maya held the herbs tightly so they wouldn't spill.

The moon was out, yin filled the world.
The stars shone bright and snowflakes gently swirled.

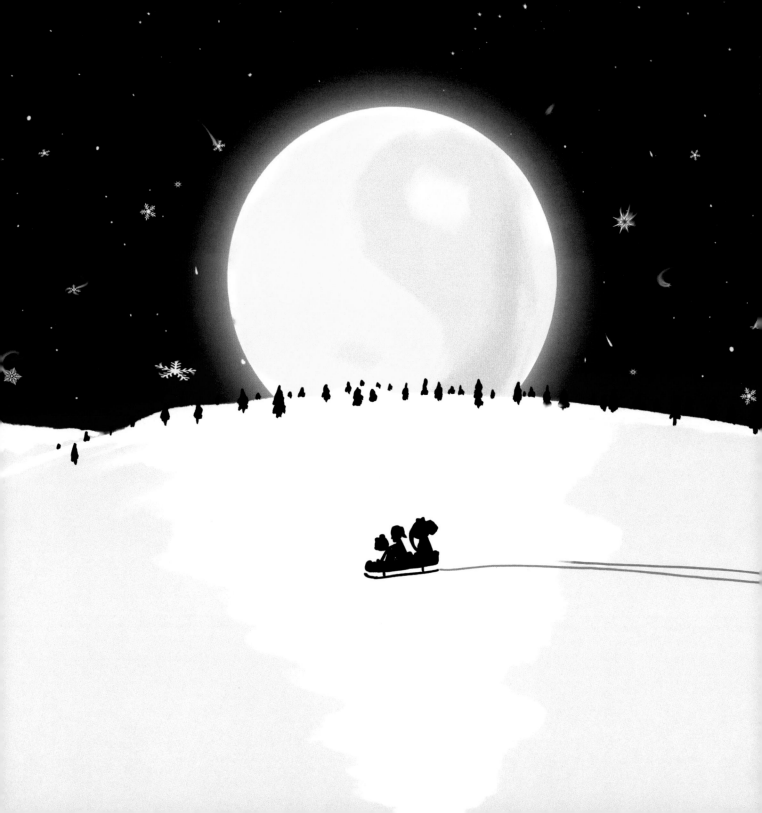

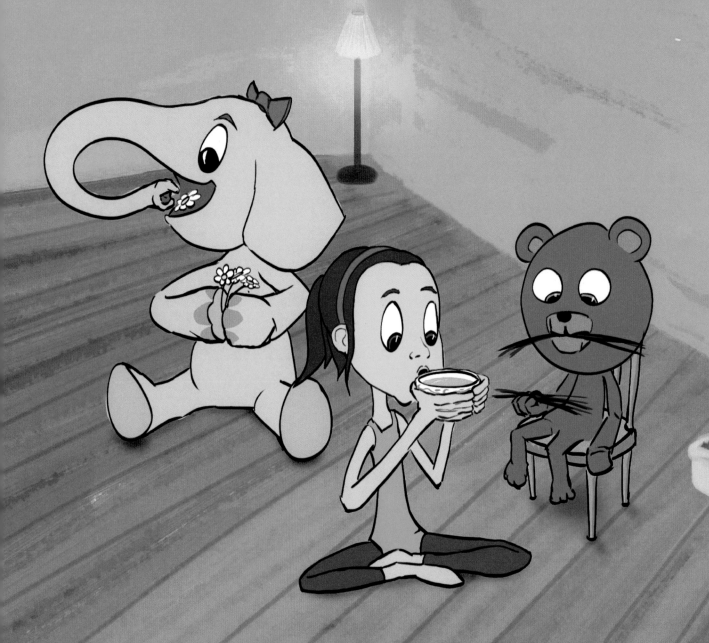

At home, Maya drank her herbs nice and warm.
Her friends had theirs in a more natural form.

Maya's **trust** in her **body's wisdom** was growing.
She slept **soundly** that night—**calm energy** flowing.

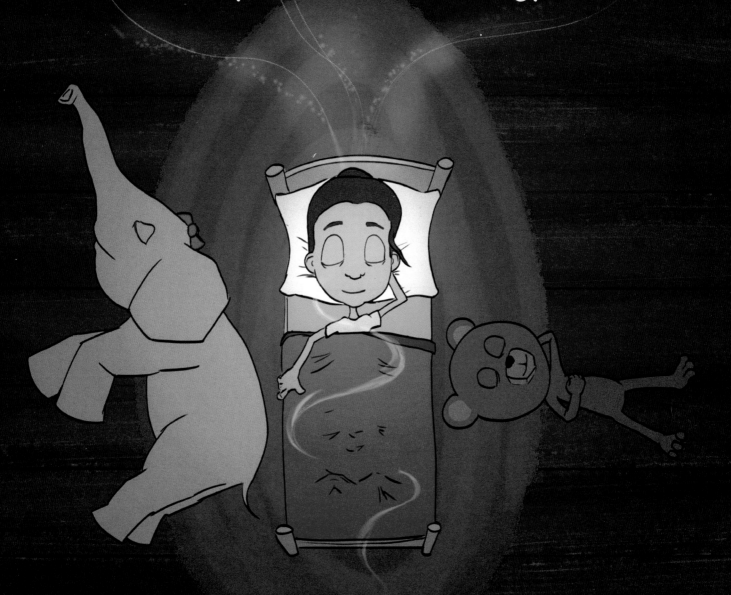

When she woke the next morning,

Her body felt strong.

The sun was shining

And the birds sang their song.

The three friends went out to play.

After all, it was the yang time of day.

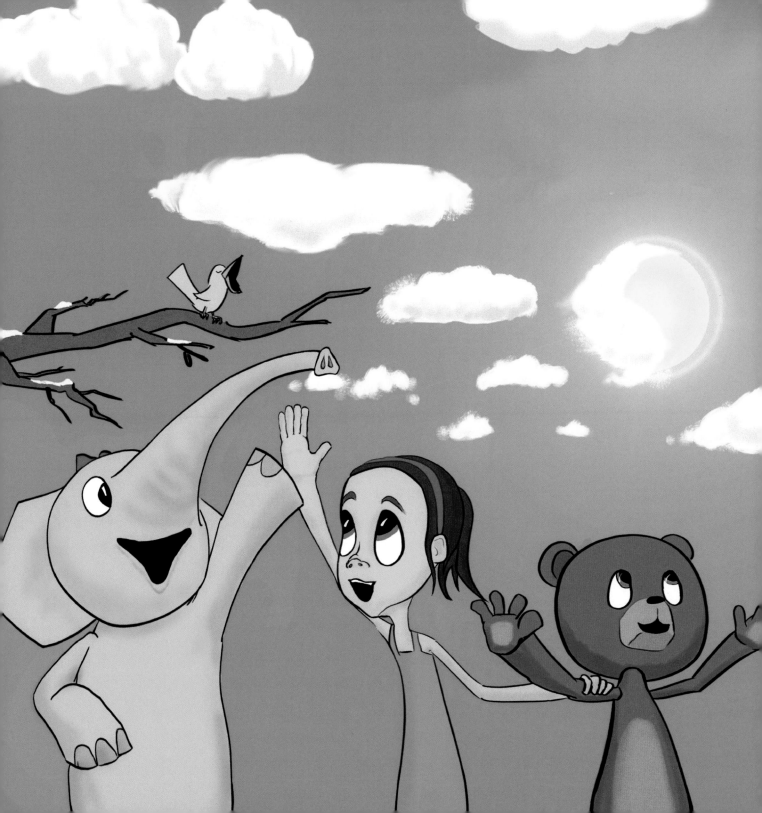

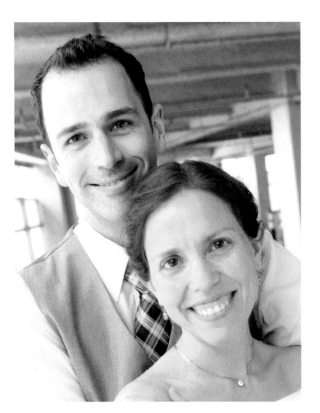

Samara White, LAc - *Author*

Samara has been working in the health and wellness field for years, and is a licensed acupuncturist and craniosacral practitioner with a master's degree from the Seattle Institute of Oriental Medicine. She was inspired to write this book to communicate the concepts of Chinese medicine in a fun and educational way that kids and adults alike can enjoy.

Troy White - *Illustrator*

Troy has been drawing all of his life, and works as a designer, communicating with imagery. He used his craft to make illustrations that bring these characters and concepts to life in a magical way.